THE ILLUSION OF AGE

The Fallacy of Decline

by
Seaon Ducoté

PublishAmerica
Baltimore

First printing

ISBN: 1-4137-0163-9
PUBLISHED BY PUBLISHAMERICA, LLLP
www.publishamerica.com
Baltimore

Printed in the United States of America

The Fountain of Youth lies within. To reach it one must realize and understand that we were all Made In The Image and Likeness of God.

We are not bound by "time," or body. We are Spirit! Think it and believe it and watch the changes.

Contents

Introduction

"The most beautiful thing we can experience is the mysterious. It is the source of all true art and science. He to whom this emotion is a stranger, who can no longer pause to wonder and stand rapt in awe, is as good as dead: his eyes are closed." —Albert Einstein

The mental and physical process society refers to as "aging" is as complex as our search for God, and in truth that is exactly what it is. Every stage of life is our God given opportunity to awaken to our full potential of spirituality, talents, dreams and goals. It is a process that should never be viewed with limits. It is our life and how long we choose to linger in each stage should not be determined by anyone but the "self." And certainly not measured within the limits of years lived.

The process towards realization of our true beingness, viewed in metaphysical beliefs, is timeless. But to many Americans, it is limited to one lifetime. Whatever your belief, the process of aging for an estimated 55 million Americans 50 and over, has descended into mediocrity and social and economic segregation.

From the age of 40, we are programmed to believe that we are "over the hill." At 50 years, the American business of aging begins. Mailboxes are flooded with brochures soliciting burial insurance, will kits, senior discounts, retirement communities, and nursing home insurance. Suddenly, we awake to find that we have become an American commodity.

Our search for God is not a guarantee that we will have a full understanding and realization of spiritual truths at age 20 or 100. But it is our human right and privilege to search without social and economic limitations. It is ludicrous to believe that men or women, of any age, can be trapped into believing that they have a time limit on their achievements, dreams and their search to have all that life can offer. George Bernard Shaw once said, *"This is the true joy in life, the being used for a purpose recognized by yourself as a mighty one."*

Each stage of our life process revolves around our choice to conform to mass thought or cultivate our own belief system. And herein lies the problem for most Americans. To be accepted in America, you must be counted as part of the American conformity of mass thought and deed. Ironically, as birthdays creep nearer to the 40th year, a vast majority of Americans feel their dream *to be all they can be* coming to an end. They feel they have no choice but to accept the journey *over the hill.*

The thought seeps into the mind and binds the spirit. Women live in fear of what they will become, who will want them, and who will leave them. Men often take their refuge from the thought of decline by giving more thought to the past than possibilities for the future. But both find they are in a whirlpool being sucked to the bottom of society.

The price of courage to be yourself without the stigma

of a number is not easy. We are all children of God with the responsibility to be our best in body and soul. But looking young and being the best at what you do will not save you from the social stigma of being labeled "old" at the earthly age of 50. So, what's so bad about being labeled a "senior?" It is a label that is measured by the word "old." It mentally separates you from the mainstream of life.

We speak of human rights, civil rights, equal rights, women's rights, discrimination, and the crime of segregation of the African/American and Native American race. But the largest segment of our society that lives with the stigma of family, social, economic discrimination and segregation, is the American population 50 years and over. Ironically, they are their own worst enemy as they walk in silent acceptance of their fate.

It is my hope that this book will give you insight into the illusion of aging. How you choose to use these facts and personal stories will determine your choice of "letting" or letting go of the concept of aging. The exit out of this concept requires a sense of adventure, determination and grace. It means celebrating your birth as the day that your mother gave you birth. It means living your life without numbers — forever free.

Part One
The Inspiration To Our Demise

Beaker or flagon, or bowl or jar,
Clumsy or slender, coarse or fine;
However the potter may make or mar,
All were made to contain the wine:
Should we seek this one ... or that one shun
When the wine which gives them their worth is one.
—an ancient Sufi utterance.

In 1993 the news media branded America's small nursing homes as breeding grounds for abuse among the "blue collar" elderly. Investigative reporters provided network television with hidden camera videos revealing traumatized residents strapped in wheelchairs, roaches scurrying across open bedsores, and aides caught in the act of physical abuse. Attorneys, nationwide, quickly launched advertising campaigns soliciting families who suspected nursing home abuse of a loved one.

Over the years, we have been periodically bombarded with these traumatic stories, but the psycho-social structure of personality types living in nursing and assisted living facilities still remains as the unspoken and unrecognized core of mental and physical abuse in facilities, large or small.

The separation of the "older" generation from a new and modern society began to evolve at the close of World War II. A new beginning in world trade and the rising popularity of television opened unlimited business opportunities throughout major cities. The American

Dream suddenly became a reality. Middle age parents in rural areas began to witness the exodus of young men and women opting for a more lucrative city lifestyle. As the 60's dawned, product demand opened doors for women in the workplace and slowly closed the doors to family home care of aging relatives. It was a new America — a youth oriented America no longer in need of maintaining reliance on the family counsel of the elder "core" parents.

Nursing homes, soon became the answer to relieving busy families of a responsibility, once readily accepted by adult children. The new American concept of aging was packaged and marketed to a busy youth oriented world that believed that the age groups are happier around "their own kind." This convenient and lawful idea of segregation quickly put profiteers into action with small poorly staffed facilities, projecting a home-type atmosphere that appeared to ensure loved ones a longer life span.

The birth of the nursing home was, in fact, a progressive idea of caring for the elderly who needed 24 hour observation and care, but it was never designed to fulfill mental or emotional needs. The nursing home operation was, and still is, designed as a low budget/ high profit operation. Psycho-social problems that are too expensive, or complicated, to resolve, are ignored allowing thousands of residents to yearly succumb to the mental trauma of emotional abandonment.

Modern medicine has only recently come to the conclusion that the process of aging is as good as our thoughts, exercise, food, and vitamin intake. It is now a scientific fact that, negative thoughts, unresolved goals, family issues, guilt and anger, contribute to chemical poisons and neurosis, while vitamin deficiencies foster senility and bone deterioration.

Ironically, facts relating to the reaction of negative thoughts were truths revealed by religious sects from the ancient Vedic writings to the late 1800 teachings of Mary Baker Eddy's Christian Science. In 1901 The Theosophical Society in America published a small book entitled, *Thought Forms* by Annie Besant and C.W. Leadbeater. This book, has proved to be mysteriously ahead of it's time, in revealing how the actions and reactions of our thoughts and the thoughts of others affect our body and the world around us.

Negative thought forms, regarding aging, have now taken our society to an all time low in self esteem and dignity. Because of our society's obsession with youth, women as young as age 40 fear loneliness in later years unless they opt for a face-lift. Women's rights are now challenged to embark on a new frontier. The right of natural appearance in the home and workplace.

Men severely wrinkled, graying and bald are accepted in high profile career positions, as well as marriages to women 30 or 40 years their junior. It is a serious and sorrowful fact that the majority of women reaching the age of 50, no longer feel needed or accepted in our youth obsessed society.

In a critical moment of compiling this manuscript — a moment when the verbal communication needed to explain the drama of aging seemed frozen in futility — a simple answer appeared from within the stems of a barren

Hibiscus bush, rescued from a neighboring trash container. Rescuing plants is a hobby that presents my soul with more pleasure than purchasing a sturdy specimen in full bloom. There has always been something quite metaphysical, and at times, magical, in the ritual of their revival.

Sparking the dormant energy within a plant (not unlike the same process with the human spirit) is a process of catering to the wrinkle and frown of limb and leaf. It is about discovering the level of their trauma and delight.

Some plants prefer to be alone — others are more social and thrive in a crowd of other limbs and leaves. Some like morning sun — others afternoon — daily watering or weekly watering. And then there is the human problem; It is a scientific fact that humans vibrate with negative or positive energy. These vibrations can literally kill a plant or generate growth. And so, the process of nurturing the traumatized soul of a plant is not unlike that of a human spirit.

In this particular instance, I had placed the pitiful pot of sticks in my window, atop a small pedestal. There I faithfully watered it over a period of three weeks. I chose to keep the existing soil and refrain from inserting any chemicals. It's revival solely depended on the support energy of belief, water, light, soft music, and most importantly, the flourishing auras of 14 healthy plants.

One evening, as I put my notes aside, I casually glanced toward the Hibiscus and found to my joy and amazement a belief system manifested. Tiny tips of leaf growth protruded from top to bottom of every limb. My much needed analogy of aging appeared before my eyes and suddenly the subject of aging and the once barren plant became one-in-the-same.

It was apparent to me, at that moment, that trauma, disease, positive and negative environments, lead us in and out of seasons of personal beauty and appearances of failure and dying. And just like the barren plant, our continued growth or **creation** depends on the belief system around, and within, us. We literally, live, act, and breath in unison with the vibrations — energy forces within our personal environment.

Lives void of a passionate purpose, often grow weary, frightened and bitter. As spiritual beings, we eventually may discover that it is not enough to live for the approval of others, or to seek a sense of security solely in the accumulation of possessions. Reaching our 40th, 50th, 60th, 70th, and 80th year of life often requires that we recreate our self outwardly and inwardly. It can be a period of fulfillment and spiritual renewal, or the beginning of martyrdom.

Bertrand Russell once said, *"It is preoccupation with possessions, more than anything else, that prevents us from living freely and nobly."* On a bus trip from Washington state to Texas I had the pleasure to meet a woman in her 76th year of life. Our conversation touched on many subjects before she inquired about my destination. At that point, we traded stories of our reason for travel. Sarah was married with a small home in Idaho. Upon reaching her 74th birthday, she began to feel a mental and physical drain and was simply "going through the motions" of living. But Sarah had a good role model. She remembered her mother doing charity work until the day she passed away in her 95th year of life.

"When I remembered how happy mother was to the end, I knew I was wasting my love and experiences sitting around thinking my life was over."

Sarah decided to minister to homeless shelters across America. She now rides the bus from one direction to another, periodically stopping in towns or cities that she feels "called" to preach.

I will always remember the glow of happiness in the eyes of this tiny woman who found a purpose in which to live. Sarah is only one of many I have met who have chosen to ignore the social stigma and limits of the American "senior label." Unfortunately, the majority of our 35 million Americans over the earthly age of 40 buy into the concept of a social numbering system that dictates the onset of their decline and segregation. They live in fear and depression of their changing body — forgetting the power that lies within their spirit.

I have spent most of my life working in the Arts as a writer and visual artist, and as in any phase of the Arts, each individual is the sum total of their talent. Age is never considered or feared. Like the creation of a fine painting, its maturity and beauty appears with each stroke of life. And each stroke is a celebration.

Year after year, I have observed friends and family, outside of the Arts, turn to the fear and thought of decline as they approach their 40thth year. At 50 years, their mailbox became the messenger of mental doom — like red hot lava with a continuous flow of advertisements for burial insurance, retirement plans, nursing home insurance and Will kits.

I began to take pity on those caught up in this insidious sentence of mental death. I then began to understand how my 16 years of metaphysical training had altered my state of consciousness. Aging — to me, did not exist. I was content in the knowledge of "I Am." I didn't understand how society could overlook the fact that our conception of time had been totally displaced by Einstein when he proved that time is relative with the capacity to speed up or slow down. It seemed so clear to me that I controlled my own time and determined the speed of my deterioration in accordance with my own thoughts, as well as, my reactions to another's thoughts. It became obvious to me that our fears and life issues literally create our demise.

After two years of thought on the subject and the graduation of my daughter, I decided to go back to college to secure a degree in social work. My plan was to enter into the nursing home field as combination Social Worker/ Activity Director. Looking back, I am now amazed that I believed in any possibility to heal and inspire those locked in the confines of a commercial belief system of decline.

When I began serving my social work internship in a Texas nursing and assisted living facility, it soon became apparent that the residents retained the same emotional needs as anyone at any stage of life experience. Life's little joke! Our emotional needs continue on and are still very much alive and in place, no matter what state of decline one has developed. The need to be touched, held, and to fall in love are just as important to the heart and soul as when the body and mind were operative.

After serving a very emotional 14-month internship I realized the tremendous need to educate others to live without the stigmas, labels, and aging categories. I also realized that it was an educational process that should begin as early as possible in an individual's life. Unfortunately, I wasn't prepared for the social and economic challenges that I would face in order to demonstrate and begin this work.

I have since realized that my belief in the illusion of age is my choice, and no matter how many times I have proved it to my self, or inspired others to take responsibility in dispelling their own illusion, I seem to be forever caught in the frustration of watching society's determination to hold to the idea that "older" means weaker and wiser.

Recently, my boyfriend, younger in life experience than I, leaned lovingly into my ear and whispered, "You are wiser, because you are older." I laughed at such a silly but accepted notion. Was this the problem society created for older women dating younger men? Is this why it is much more accepted for an older man to be with a younger woman? Is it because an older man is thought to be wiser because he is older, therefore women should be with someone wiser than they? Wrinkles, loss of hair — all go with the wiser man's image of wisdom.

The "older" woman, involved with a younger man — even if she is youthful in appearance, enters a questionable area in our society. The thought that she could have fallen in love with a younger man's personality, or attributes is laughable in most families or social circles. And more often than not, the consensus points to sex as being her motivation. Eventually, her lover or companion also becomes questionable in his own eyes. It is a rare man or woman that can stand strong in society and realize that love has no limits in time and space. It just is and should be enjoyed for as long as it works for both.

Through trial and error and experimentation, I have found that we are victims of our limited beliefs in the transformation of mind and body and spirit. At times, someone breaks out of the norm: a concert pianist at nine years, a university graduate at 16 years, a woman of 96 years, sky diving, etc. But breaking out of the limited life box that mankind calls "normal" demands a price in our society.

Americans fear or resent their later years — programed by society's fear of aging as the door to death. This belief brings a sense of social abandonment — *no longer wanted or needed* in society because it is thought that they have reached their peak — seen their day. Women, more than men, turn to face lifts, lip and nose make-overs. But the fear of age cannot be cut away.

You may smooth your character lines, peel, and stretch until you obtain the accepted appearance for someone 30 or 40 years in experience. You may attract men 20 years younger, but if the relationship evolves, eventually, there is always the consideration of his fears for the future of a long term relationship. Corrective surgery does not erase the fatal view of age that most people carry within.

The infamous birthday that puts us "over the social

hill," looms in the shadows like some distant funeral march. Who will die before the other? Who will wrinkle first? Will I be embarrassed by kissing a woman or man that is not as smooth as I? Our thoughts on the *age factor*, regarding relationships, revolve around appearance more than love of soul and spirit, or the qualities a person can bring to our life.

In the early sixties, my uncle married a woman 15 years his senior. They were the gossip of the family. He was 25 and she was 40. The family was sure it was destined to doom. But the marriage grew and blossomed until the day of her Passing in her at 79th year.

Our society constantly falls suspect to any union of two people with an age difference. Men are afraid to love an older woman because of family and social embarrassment. But because a man can generate children to a late stage of life, it is accepted when an elder man marries a younger woman. Are we talking about discrimination here, or simply, spiritual ignorance?

I have had two major love affairs with men 16 to 24 years younger in life experience than I. The problem was never our compatibility, but ultimately, their fear of "what people would think." The social stigma of age — what one *should* act like — look like, upon arriving at a specific number of birthdays — all takes precedence over *love*.

To be forever young — to experience and be interested in life without limits of age is to be considered an oddball, irresponsible, immature. Ironically, to be attracted to or involved with a younger, or elder man or woman is no greater gamble than involvement with someone in the early adult stage of life. Relationships of any type are our ***own Deliberate Creation, as is our resignation to limitation, based on a number.***

One year ago I met a man that was kind and seemed to have a special quality of character that I enjoyed being around. I had just moved to the mountains of Western Washington. I had lived in a large city most of my life and had reached a time in my life where I needed to challenge myself. Our meeting came through a neighbor who recommended his work in home repairs.

Over a period of a month we became friends. I had a younger girlfriend that I thought would be a good match for him, but she didn't seem interested and he was cooling off on the idea. One night after sharing dinner, he turned to me and told me that I was the one who had won his heart. I was shocked. I knew we had an attraction for each other, but I was still trying to get past a broken relationship from two years prior. It too, had been a man much younger than I.

I sent Lynn home that night, but as the days went by and our conversations intensified, we eventually became involved in an affair that seemed to supply both of us with joy. Lynn was 22 years younger than I, but for ten months we shared meals, made love, and shared stories of our life.

He had asked my age in the beginning of our affair. I tried to explain my views and metaphysical beliefs on the subject and that I never revealed my earthly age. The subject was never brought up again until ten months later. During those ten months, Lynn was my mentor. He was tough and wise in the strategy of survival in the mountains of the Northwest. He taught me to handle guns, make camp fires, hunt and fish. It was an exciting time for me in every way. Eventually the mystery of the forest slowly took on a harder meaning. I was learning to be tough in a tough environment.

I could literally feel myself changing within. I lost weight, felt strong, younger and in control. It was something I had never felt in the city. I was at a peak in physical beauty and performance at the earthly stage of 62. Ironically, the area men and women guessed my age at around 44 years. At last, I was proving everything I believed about the illusion of age. My formula, for years, was to daily tell myself that I was 37, (a number in Tibetan belief meaning *eternal*). I had visualized this number for so long that I truly felt it — believed it. It was obvious to me that I had found the secret and broken the code of decline.

But, as quickly as the relationship began, it seemed to end. One night while sharing a meal, Lynn became serious — somewhat angry. He insisted on knowing my age. I refused to tell him and he walked out. What had happened? We had no intentions of marriage, so why was this an issue. I had never lied about my age.

I just refrained from revealing it. Why was I being forced into telling him? I knew if I told him that he would never be able to handle such a large age difference with himself — or with his friends.

The next day I violated my spiritual values, which I refer to as unplugging from my God source. I called Lynn and told him that I was only ten years older. I had instantly unplugged myself from an "ageless"status to the mindset of the masses. I made the choice to be 48 years "old" to save a relationship with a man who had no knowledge of metaphysics, nor did he understand my work or mission.

I was now living in the same fear of age as I had always told others to ignore. I had become someone that I no longer knew. Why didn't I just stand up to the pressure and hang onto my belief of being ageless? At least, I would have ended the relationship with my dignity and principals in tact.

Lynn was satisfied with the number until the age factor surfaced again. Obsessed to know if I was telling the truth, he went through my wallet while I was in another room. He found my drivers license and found the answer. For two weeks he said nothing about it, but looking back on those two weeks, he seemed to have a different softness in the way he treated me.

It was interesting the way he announced his knowledge of my secret. It was in the middle of a football game. He turned to me with a smile on his face and said, "I know when you were born." I was stunned. I tried to discuss it, but he laughed and told me we would talk about it in a year. I had no idea what that meant, but out of fear I didn't push the issue. I felt a violation of my person, principals, and belief. I had allowed someone to lead me out of my own world and throw me head first into their own beliefs and limitations.

I knew it was the end of our childlike playfulness. I was so afraid that the longer he thought about it, the whole relationship would develop according to his programming of "age." Would I become the "granny in the forest" that he would visit when he wasn't busy? I had come out of my cocoon — allowing myself to look and be 20 years younger. Now I was forced to view age from his reality. I had lost control of my reality and entered his illusion.

"Pandora's Box" opened. Why was I trying to prove my ability to be as young as I wanted to be to a man who knew nothing about metaphysics or any of the healing arts. My position was to teach, not oblige his beliefs.

His need to know outweighed the need to "just be" and enjoy our relationship. Am I still age 37? Yes. Will I ever be able to go back to my eternally young vision in my mind? Yes, I walk in it daily. The truth is that I was hanging onto a number, not the symbol, and when challenged, I simply chose another number instead of holding to my belief.

The experience was a "wake-up-call" for me. I was living the ageless concept on the outside, but inside, I still relied on the self hypnosis of associating a number with eternal youth. I am now, thankful for the adjustment that I have had to make in order to be true to myself. I can never escape the amount of earthly years I have lived, but I have risen above it in the knowledge that the number is not who I am.

What happened to Lynn? We are 2,500 miles away from each other, but still maintain a friendship. There is a strange magic between us in that we have learned to respect, not change, each other's beliefs. I think we are both in awe of our survival tactics — especially mine.

Part Two
Through The Looking Glass

Sweet life ...
Into the looking glass
I walk,
Following some sweet illusion,
Bumping my head on,
Before and after,
Looking, looking,
For a way in or out,
Until, at last,
I see ...
The reflection of life
Is me ... the inspiration
to my demise.

My first knowledge of nursing homes came in 1965. My mother received a telephone call from her two sisters in a neighboring state. The sisters lived in the same city as my grandmother, often surprising her with unannounced visits. On one occasion, the sisters had found my grandmother of 80 years in her backyard picking peaches, clad in her underwear and slip.

She had pulled a chair next to the trunk of the tree and lifted herself up into the fork of the trunk. Was she senile? No! Was she demented or insane? No! She claimed that she wanted to feel the warm sun on her shoulders and added that she was perfectly capable of picking her own peaches. Mamie had always been an active, creative woman. She was doing what she had always done. But her daughters decided that she was becoming senile — not acting like a woman her "age."

Shortly after the incident, we received a telephone call informing my mother that they had admitted grandmother to a nursing home *for her own safety*. My mother was horrified that she had not been consulted. But instead of taking action to rescue her mother, she chose never to speak to her sisters again. Grandmother was in perfect health, but lived only 17 months after being admitted. During those 17 months she made numerous attempts to escape. Eventually she gave up, went to bed one day, and let go of any recognition of family and friends. It was easier for her to just pass away then to be imprisoned.

As fast as peeling a banana the disoriented, crippled, and weak are stripped of self-esteem, hopes, dreams, motivation, and desire. Thousands of elderly men and women are continually taken out of the family "fold" and placed in the custody of profiteers and an overworked, (and often uneducated), staff. Few adult children take the time to explore the possibilities of a home healthcare program. In perspective, this cannot be considered unusual since few Baby Boomers experienced early childhood development in a home where parents were the caretakers for a grandparent who was still considered a valuable part of the family nucleus.

One major factor in today's society is that most adult children usually have unresolved issues or personality conflicts that make the thought of bringing an ailing elderly parent into their home, a nightmare. The result of this failure to resolve family issues is apparent as many of our social and industrial pioneers are admitted to a luxury facility to await death, caged in an emotional state of trauma, rejection, and lack of purpose. Our warriors of experience and wisdom have become a cartoon of the "American Dream."

There is a joke among nursing home staff. "If they're not dying when they come in, they soon will be." Unfortunately, it is more of a reality than a joke. When the disabled or dying elder is taken out of their home environment, they have then lost the last thread of security and purpose for living.

Metaphysically, the event society terms "death" is the spiritual transition from one dimension to another. And according to clergy, prophets, and eastern beliefs, the transition or "passing on" is as important as our birth. But even in the most luxurious of facilities, this moment is often experienced without the vigil of family, or staff.

The major problem experienced by nursing and assisted living residents is depression. This is not difficult to understand if you can imagine how you would feel if your family appeared in your home or hospital room to announce *their* plan for your on-going *well being*. The following scenario was described to me by a new resident during my tenure as an activity director:

Smiling faces try to assure you that you will be much safer and happier in a place where you can have friends and activities to keep you busy. Suddenly you feel overwhelming fear rise to your throat. Your mind races for a solution. Suspicion mounts! You feel caught. No longer in control of your life.

But the faces around you keep smiling sweetly, relating that it's for your own good. You want to fight, argue with their decision, but the guilt of being a burden to your family keeps your thoughts silent. You feel worthless and embarrassed. Everyone seems to be talking over and around you as if you're not in the room. You wonder how your life could have come to such an end.

Then the day arrives. You are ushered into a hotel-like setting. Everyone is smiling, except the residents, as they roam through the halls and lobby. Like a child entering daycare for the first time, you are rigid with fear and denial. You know it must be a mistake. It's all a mistake. You are lead to a freshly painted room with a bed, chair and T.V. You're seated in a soft recliner while the family makes small talk. Then the moment comes. They must leave, but they say they will come by tomorrow. You want to scream, "Let me go with you, I won't be a bother!" You want to get on your knees and beg, but you smile and say your goodbyes.

Depression is usually inevitable and often psyhcotrophic drugs are administered to help with mental anguish. But the drugs leave the resident disoriented and soon the battle to find a reason for living becomes a mute point within the pain of abandonment. How long the drugs will be administered depends on how well the resident adjusts to their surroundings. The truth is that very few residents find solace in such an environment.

According to the U.S. Department of Health and Human Services, depression in the elderly is helped by:

A. Give the resident hope for the future.

B. Talk about things they have enjoyed in the past andcan realistically look forward to in the future.
C. Let the resident talk about their dark feelings and offer sympathetic support without doing everything for him or her.

In both "A" and "B" reference is made to the need for emotional reliance on the future. Surely they jest! At this stage, all possibilities of any purpose in life has been eliminated. And the mental welfare has now been assigned to an $8 to $12 dollar an hour Activity Director.

Nursing and assisted living facilities can be a haven for many if the purpose was to create a daily "purpose" to those in their care. But the majority of activities are mindless trivia because of the facility's inability to deal with life issues, family, and mental illness. Because of this factor, any remaining mental capabilities soon deteriorate as the resident slips into a member of the facility's collective consciousness.

The collective consciousness of these facilities is not unlike the individual personalities of a dysfunctional family.

A. Family Heroes: Responsible; follows rules and seeks approval.
B. The Family Clown: Immature; fragile; distracting; tries to be cute.
C. The Victim: Hostile; self-pity; charming; rigid values; manipulative.
D. The Martyr: Physically sick; sarcastic; passive; super-responsible.

E. The Scapegoat: The rule-breaker; defiant; hostile.
F. The Angel: Lost child; shy; quiet; attaches self to things, not people; solitary.

The staff operates through a parent/child type of relationship with the Administrator as the acting mother or father image of the family. Hate, greed, sexual deviation, and fantasy become intertwined to the point whereby the only purpose for the sane is to establish a friendship (a type of comic relief) with the demented.

Few volunteers have been properly educated to this underlying consciousness and are often shocked when they realize that most of the residents are not mentally challenged. The trained and dedicated volunteer will eventually recognize the cruel stream of resident consciousness empowered by the "dysfunctional" list of personalities.

An example of this type of cruelty among residents is reflected in the following incident observed during my internship at a luxury nursing and assisted living facility:

Alma was a 90 year elderly woman who used a walker with an attached basket, as a purse, to carry her trinkets from room to room. Her timid smile and pleasant manner gave new volunteers the impression that she was a lovely little lady in excellent shape for her age. But after participating in the facility's Bingo night they realized the truth.

Alma's memory can best be described visually, as having the same qualities as a weathered limestone in the rain. Small amounts of rain collect in the tiny pockets for a short period of time, but within minutes dissolve into the cracks and crevices. One evening, during an intense Bingo game with 20 other residents, Alma looked up from her card in total confusion. Tears welled in her eyes as she yelled at me from across the room.

"I can't use this card! Something is wrong with it."

Silence engulfed the room. Everyone turned to me with disgusted faces. Bingo was as serious to them as sitting at a Las Vegas Blackjack table betting your last dollar.

"Alma," I asked, "what could be wrong with your card?"

"The numbers you're calling are not on this card."

The silence ruptured into hysterical laughter. Alma quickly seated herself, retreating from the cruel laughter. Her face a tangled line of confusion. I walked to her table and apologized for giving her such a bad card. She smiled, put the card in her basket, and left the room through a maze of complaints and cruel insults. Alma was the "lost child" — the angel lost in an alien world

In order to survive the emotional trauma, the ailing or abandoned elder must develop survival skills. Often these skills are no more than significant types of personality disorders developed in the absence of "purpose" and family ties. Or possibly, they have carried a disorder, unnoticed and unresolved, throughout life.

~~~
~~~

Myrtle was a prime example of someone that used her survival skills to adapt to her environment. She was 55 years of age and diagnosed with acute hypochondria and obsessive/compulsive disorder. Her condition was not under the supervision of a psychiatrist when admitted. Her family physician had prescribed sedatives and suggested locating her on the skilled nursing floor, rather than the assisted living section. It was a selfish course of action that allowed a prominent family to remain safe from the embarrassment of seeking psychiatric attention for their family member.

One of the items that was not allowed in the skilled nursing section was aerosol spray, but Myrtle, with the aides knowledge, had several types hidden in her room. Myrtle was fully aware that she was an embarrassment to her family and rarely received visits. This caused her to devise her own type of in-house family security.

Because she was a resident of the skilled nursing unit, she was assigned a wheelchair, which she used in much the same way as we use a shopping cart. Although, she had no history of criminal behavior before being admitted, her need to somehow control a small portion of her existence resulted in a type of sociopath activity by stealing from women she had befriended. Her stolen items were given to the aides in her unit in exchange for favors.

Periodically, the facility would have surprise visits from state inspectors. Their visits usually caused aides to scurry to check rooms and their assigned areas before the inspectors entered their unit. On such a morning, Myrtle saw the tension mounting in her care givers. Immediately, she set out to warn each floor, including the kitchen staff. Myrtle reacted in much the same way that abused children react when their family secrets are in danger of being exposed. Myrtle was typical of the "martyr" personality in the dysfunctional family. The family protector.

~~~

Benny had been admitted with Multi-Infarct Dementia. In this disorder a series of cerebral interruptions of the blood supply to areas of the brain destroy neurons throughout expanding brain regions. The progressive loss of cells leads to brain atrophy and behavioral impairment that ultimately mimic Dementia of the Alzheimer type.

Benny was the nursing home family clown. His slim, agile figure would sway, twirl, and dance gracefully down the hallway and dining room. At times he would stand idly by at the nurses station, smiling and commenting in low, soft nonsensical words that only held meaning to Benny.

During special nursing home events, holidays, and birthdays, Benny would rise to the music, never bothering to find a partner. There would be a combination of jeers, laughter, and applause for his joyful "moves." Benny was comparable to a court jester in the minds of the residents and staff. He could not converse in an intelligible manner, but found gestures and facial expressions to relate his simple messages of love and frustration.
~~~

Every resident portrays a role in the collective consciousness of the facility. As with any town, community, school, church, or organization, the negative or positive element will either foster love and progress, or discrimination and decline. The community of residents within the nursing home is also regulated by the same unspoken factor.

Nursing, and assisted living facilities are islands in the sea of society. The residents are rarely there by choice, but like shipwrecked victims, they have been thrown into an alien environment that often leaves them feeling helpless, lonely, and without purpose. And as with any age group, stranded on an island, their choices in filling their emotional and physical needs become limited. Friendships, and physical attractions begin to evolve with partners that would, otherwise, be unthinkable when they were in the mainstream of society.

~~~

And so it was with Leroy, an active 92 year, six foot, three inch, elder with a unique ability to motivate others. He had lived the American Dream and would quickly let everyone know how undeserving he was of all his good fortune. I had always thought he was joking, but later learned that he carried much grief and guilt for the pain he had caused his wife and daughter. Pain that was never resolved.

Leroy, the son of a Texas vegetable farmer, began his
~~~

career in the Spring of 1922, graduating with a degree in business from Rice University, priding himself in being one of the first graduating classes. He immediately moved to Houston where he started the first fast food restaurant, becoming a pioneer in the industry, and President of its statewide association.

The "perfect life" continued for 63 years. He retired in 1965 with a winter home in Colorado, a mansion in Houston, and major investments worldwide. For the next 20 years Leroy and his wife lived the life of an extended vacation, traveling the world. Then, at age 83, Leroy was faced with caring for a wife diagnosed with Alzheimer Disease. The American Dream became a nightmare.

After two years, Leroy could no longer care for his wife. At that point his children, then in their late 40's, stepped into the picture. The businesses were sold, along with the mansion in Houston. When a suitable nursing/assisted living facility was located, Leroy refused to abandon his wife. He decided to live in the assisted living quarters two floors away from his wife.

I was introduced to Leroy in the summer of 1993, as the new Activity Director, responsible for the psycho/social well-being of 92 residents. He had lived on the same floor and in the same room for seven years without taking part in any of the activities offered. His daily routine for seven years was to sit in his room until 3:00 p.m, then walk down the hall to the elevator for his visit with his wife. She had lost recognition of him several years prior, but still, he would sit for an hour talking to her and pleading for forgiveness into the glazed eyes, void of love or emotion.

He would always leave with tears streaming down his face, head bent, retreating to the darkness of his room. This is how I found him on my second day of employment. I had been visiting with each resident, encouraging them to share their "likes" and dislikes with me. The interviews consisted of talking about their past and getting the personal information I needed to create individualized activities.

When I entered Leroy's room, I could see a dark image seated in the corner chair. I stood frozen, uncertain as to whether I should invade his privacy with a rude flash from the light switch.

"Leroy, are you napping?"

"Come in honey. I'm not asleep."

Immediately, I switched on the light. I felt like "Dorothy," exposing the Wizard of Oz. Leroy quickly wiped his red eyes with an oversized red handkerchief. He was not the type of man that one could comfortably picture in a mood of humble sorrow. For the next three months, I visited Leroy daily, bringing him puzzles, books and games, but they would always remained untouched.

My visits with Leroy were always a concerned pleasure for me. He would always smile and hold out his hand to me. "Honey, come give me a hug." Leroy was always asking for hugs from females in every stage of life. Sometimes he would steal a "pat" or two from the rear of a pretty nurse, or unsuspecting resident.

One evening, after the ten o'clock news, he exposed himself to the lady across the hall. When he was brought before the Administrator the following morning, he declared that he was only responding to the lady's habit of parading to the nurses station in her nightgown. He thought she was flirting with him.

Except for his occasional bouts of amorous behavior, Leroy was a perfectly behaved resident. The frustration, regarding my failure to inspire him to participate in activities, was mounting within myself and the Administrator. It was my job to motivate bedside, or group activities, but nothing seemed to work with Leroy.

One afternoon, while we sat visiting in his room, I noticed how much he used the word, "work." Suddenly I awoke to the need of this businessman. He loved to talk — to give advice. He had been an employer, father, and a husband. He didn't need to be entertained. He had played and entertained himself for 20 years before entering the facility.

The following morning I entered his room at nine a.m.

"It's time to go to work, Leroy."

He laughed and ask me for his usual hug. But I stepped back out of the reach of his out-stretched arms.

"Leroy, I need your help. I'm not joking about working."

He put his hands down by his sides, gazing at me with inquisitive eyes.

"There's a young man crippled with M.S. He can't use his hands or legs, Leroy. He needs a male friend. I had to put him in the ceramic class with the ladies because it's the only kind of work I have for him today. He needs a male companion to guide his hands when he paints."

I didn't wait for his answer. I quickly turned and left the

room. Fifteen minutes later, Leroy shuffled through the art room door. I was overjoyed, greeting him with a big hug. From that moment on, Leroy became the vibration and heartbeat of the class. He became the hands for Craig and the master advisor for the weak of mind. He had found a position. Every morning, at precisely nine a.m., he would appear at the art room door announcing himself to the ladies that he was there to make sure they did their work.

~~~

Deep in paperwork, updating resident activity charts, I was startled, one morning, to hear cries of help from the room across from my office. I ran across the hall to Miriam's room. She was holding tightly to each of her bed-rails while laying in a reclining position. I leaned over her small body, trying to appear calm.

"Is there something I can get for you, Miriam?"

"A clean slate, she yelled."

I quickly tried to think of something profound — some words of comfort, not thinking of asking her why she wanted a clean slate. My answer was too shallow, sounding ridiculous to a woman in her 83rd year of life with advanced stages of Parkinson's disease mixed with periodic Dementia-related delusions. "Everyday's a new beginning, Miriam."

As my smiling face peered down at her disgusted glare, her face twisted in roaring disgust. "You're stupid!" she erupted.
~~~

I had wanted to stay out of any unresolved issues and glide her into "polyannahood" and she was right. I was stupid to think that would work. I patted her hand and walked back across the hall to continue my paperwork. Suddenly, I heard her yelling and pleading for help again. Again, I rushed to her bedside. She was still laying in the same position, but holding on to the guard rails as if her life depended on them.

"Get me off this airplane!" she yelled indignantly. "I refuse to go to Miami!"

I decided to play out her delusion. "Miriam, I'll tell the pilot you want to get off. Would you like for me to do that for you?"

"Yes, of course, I would."

I turned around, as if I was talking to the pilot. "Mr. Pilot, please stop the airplane so Miriam can get off. She refuses to go any further with you." When I turned back to look at Miriam, she was glaring at me again with disgust.

"You're stupid! Who are you talking to?"

She had completely forgotten the airplane ride in a matter of seconds and appeared to have no clue that she periodically entered imaginary circumstances with imaginary players. Or were they real scenarios of her past?. Eventually, these flights of fantasy or visits to the past became more frequent. Two weeks later I was walking to the nurses station when one of the aides came running toward us with a frantic look on her face.

"I need help, fast. Miriam's laying on the floor. She's not moving."

As I ran down the hallway I was ready for the worst.

Upon entering her room I kneeled beside her.

"Miriam, can you hear me?"

Slowly, she opened her eyes. She had that disgusted look, again.

"I've been hit by a car — don't move me. Get a cop! Now!"

Fortunately, I was saved from participating in Miriam's altered state. Her daughter arrived, as she did every day.

Stephanie was a retired psychologist. She was soft spoken with long gray hair that she wore pulled back. She looked more like an artist than a psychologist — always appearing in blue jeans and loose -fitting shirts and sweaters. As I moved aside to allow Stephanie to speak with her mother, I could feel the love begin to flow between them. Not a word was said. They smiled lovingly at each other and Miriam immediately got to her feet.

In the twelve months that followed my residency I had many occasions to observe the two women. I watched several daughters visiting a parent on my floor, but the majority were very uncomfortable with each other. Some daughters were timid and others played "control" games. It wasn't difficult to see that Miriam and Stephanie were friends. There was no real conversation between them. Miriam had passed that point of ability, but their love for each other surpassed all mental barriers. Most of their visits were spent walking up and down the hallways, or to other floors. Once or twice a month, Stephanie would take Miriam home for the weekend.

Miriam's unsolved issues of life eventually ravaged her mental state to the point of violence, requiring her to be moved to a locked unit for Alzheimer victims. But nothing deterred Stephanie's display of love or daily visits. It was in the month of July when Miriam was moved to the locked unit. She asked that her mother be moved in the afternoon to give her time to decorate. When the aides brought Miriam through the door of her new room she looked like a child on Christmas morning and that is exactly what awaited her. Stephanie had simulated Christmas in July complete with stuffed animals, tiny Christmas trees and balloons. It was a work of art, as was their unspoken love for each other.

~~~

Benny and Ruth just seemed to have happened. They had never shown any interest in each other, on a daily basis, even though both had been residents on the same floor for five years. How and when Benny and Ruth fell in love was never determined. My first observance of their love for each other happened one rainy Sunday morning as I walked into the recreation room. There they stood in the middle of the empty room, arms tightly around each other's waist, quietly watching the gray winter slide down the patio doors.

From that day forth, Benny and Ruth could be seen walking the halls together, hand-in-hand. How did two people, one with an advanced stage of Dementia, and the other, in the second term of Alzheimer disease, create the communication needed for a love affair? And was it a love
~~~

affair? Yes, most likely of the purest form. A simple communion of two souls.

Ruth had been a wealthy Texas oil heiress, and ranch woman. After her husband passed away, she found solace in raising her horses. The walls of her room were filled with photographs of herself around the age of forty and fifty sitting regally on her magnificent "show" horses. She had lived a full life complete with western clothes and oil wells. Now, nearly 30 years later, she spent her days walking the halls carrying a torn photo of her favorite horse.

Benny's communication ability had been lost to his Dementia and now consisted of a hug, a kiss on the hand, and a big smile. Words were no longer possible. Could it have been possible that these basic gestures were all that was needed to capture the heart of Ruth?

Benny was a participant in my ceramic class and I would periodically deliver his work to his room. One day when I entered his room to deliver a freshly dried piece, he walked to his door and closed it quietly. We both stood motionless, a frozen smile on our faces. He smiled and walked towards me. Reaching in his pocket, he pulled out a wrinkled photograph of Ruth as a smooth skinned woman. I wondered. *Was this how he viewed her?* Could it be that age is only in the minds of the sane and healthy mind?

I thanked him for sharing the photo with me and gave him a hug. We both walked out of his room smiling like Cheshire cats. The remainder of the day he followed me everywhere, repeatedly displaying the torn photo to everyone including Ruth.

In a couple of weeks, the moments they had shared – that brief time when two spirits touched – were forgotten. Benny eventually became confused, when one day looking at the photo, he placed it in my pocket after giving me a big hug. Eventually, they both returned to their original activities – never giving each other a second glance.

~~~

The first time that I had the pleasure to meet Mildred and Lily, they were cuddled together on a love seat in the nursing home lobby. It was Sunday — sightseeing day. The two women were always first in line to board the bus that would carry them around the nearby lake. But their favorite part was the return trip — stopping at their favorite ice cream parlor.

Mildred had lived a fantasy life of a single ballerina, traveling and entertaining around the world. She had an annoying habit of trying to make everyone feel like their presence was the most important moment in her life. She would ooze with sweet compliments that seemed to flow without reason. But this was Mildred's survival tactic. It had begun in her early days of social affairs and travel. Compliments opened doors and won favors for the petite and beautiful ladies. But now, Mildred's compliments were exaggerated. She was a verbal cartoon.

Lily was the opposite. She had lived a quiet married life
~~~

and now at the earthly age of 89, she was left with one niece who visited twice a month. Her uneventful life now revolved around Mildred's compliments, flirtations, and zest for life. Lily believed every compliment and story that Mildred directed her way. Maybe that was the magic between them — the need to affirm and be affirmed.

It was my custom to invite a male vocalist or comedian to entertain in the dining area on Sunday. The women loved having a nice looking man to listen to and watch. But Mildred loved the event more than anyone in the room. She was the first to express her desire to give each entertainer a big kiss.

Lily hated Mildred's show of affection to a man and would often go back to her room in the middle of a performance. It was obvious that Lily was truly in love with Mildred. But whether or not Mildred shared the same feeling could only be determined by Mildred's desire to be by Lily's side night and day.

As the months went by, I observed that Lily didn't accompany Mildred as consistently as she had in the past. She became paranoid and argumentative with Mildred and the staff. Eventually, Lily was moved to an area in the building designed for residents needing assistance with personal care.

After Lily was moved from Mildred's floor, Lily's mental state became worse. But on Sunday, sightseeing day, Mildred would come to Lily's floor to visit. The two would compliment each other in a constant flow to the front door, into the bus and throughout the entire outing. Physical problems, suspicions, and resentment may have infringed on Lily's love for Mildred, but Mildred's devotion still made everything better for Lily, one day a week.

Part Three
Issues

The Parent
Who gave me love,
and patched my wounds.
Who laughed at my dreams,
and stopped my schemes.
Who held me close,
when all was lost.
Who kicked me out,
in the Winter frost.

The first image that comes to our minds when the subject of "senior neglect" arises, is physical abuse. But as in any relationship based on "need," the untrained, tired, or disillusioned, provider, often feels trapped. Many families opt to terminate what they perceive as an emotional horror by relieving themselves of the responsibility at whatever means is available. I do not want to give the impression that every family seeking a nursing home for their family member is abusive. Every family must evaluate their intentions based on the well-being of everyone concerned. The commitment to care for a family member in the home is usually made out of love or guilt — never out of anger. Although the on-going process may eventually cause the provider enough stress, and frustration to cause anger. If no other means of care is then available, mental or physical abuse may occur.

Unresolved issues between family members do not cease upon admittance to a nursing or assisted living facility. The following incidents are true and reflect the dangers awaiting those residents who have been abandoned, or are left under the supervision of a revengeful family member.

The most dangerous time of the day for seniors residing in a nursing facility, is between nine p.m. and six a.m. During that time, the facility is operating with a minimal staff. The average ratio of three aides to two nurses for 90 residents is a normal nightshift. Questions that should be asked by families are:

How often is each room checked during the night?

Are male nurses aides allowed to change women's diapers?

Are criminal background checks made on nurses and aides?

Abuse does not "just happen." It is a symptom of the provider's rule of "profits before safety."

~~~

Dora, a tiny woman with barely enough strength to raise her coffee cup, was a wealthy widow nearing her 90th birthday. She had one son and several nieces and nephews. It had always bothered me that this frail, quiet little woman wasn't kept in her own family home with a full-time aide, enjoying her last days in the security of family and friends. It seemed such an obvious compassion to grant a loved one who could afford the private care.

Early one Sunday morning I was approached by the
~~~

night "charge" nurse. She confided that Dora had been found at 4:30 a.m. laying naked on the floor at the foot of her bed with a gashed and broken leg. She could find no other explanation than the possibility that the helpless woman had tried to go to the restroom and tumbled off the bed.

I stared at her in amazement. We both knew how absurd that would sound to anyone who knew Dora. She had to be lifted out of bed and spend her day in a wheelchair. It was obvious that there had been foul play. I walked back to my office wondering how the report would ultimately read.

As the day unfolded, I made several comments to the supervisor that the incident should be reported to the police, but was firmly told to "let it go." The following day I noticed that one of our regular aides was absent. She was also the aide that usually attended to Dora. It was obvious at that point that the aide had been terminated for neglect. The incident was never investigated and Dora's room was quickly cleaned and painted upon her removal to the hospital.

Three months later my curiosity drove me to contact Dora's family. She had been removed from the hospital and admitted to another nursing home. Shortly thereafter, Dora passed away. I was later informed that a monetary settlement had been made by our facility to Dora's family. Unfortunately, a return on Dora's funds did nothing to help her escape a traumatic death.

~~~
~~~

Tom Black was a tall, handsome man of 78 years. He had once lived in a prestigious area near the nursing home he now resided. Mr. Black was admitted by his son and then, literally, dropped off at the front door. The paperwork had been prepared in advance, making it just a matter of getting "Dad" in the car, under the pretense of spending the night in a fine hotel until son returned from a business trip.

Tom was suffering from Dementia. He was slow in his movements and forgetful about many things that seemed unimportant to him. But he was vivid in his memory of the location of his home, family members, and the day and time of church worship.

Two weeks after Tom's arrival, he still waited anxiously for his son to return. His days were spent pleading with me to take him home or to find his lost son. But I had learned early in my employment that if I were to continue, I would refrain from bothering the families and creating a feeling of guilt. And so I treated Tom's sorrow with "white lies," long walks, and ice cream. As the weeks passed, I could see that he was withdrawing further into himself, eventually refusing to participate in any activity or conversation.

Eventually, Tom's son began to visit every other week for about 15 minutes. Unfortunately, Tom's memory found nothing to cling to during the two week intervals. No familiar sight or sounds beckoned to him from the home where he had raised his family. One Sunday afternoon, I decided to take Tom on a sightseeing tour to the lake with several other residents. I approached him with the idea and to my joy, he suddenly became excited and talkative. As I helped him into the bus he told one of the women that we were taking everyone to his house for ice cream. Based on the comment he made, I decided that I would let him ride in the front seat with me. Why not let him indulge in his fantasy of being the host, "the guy in the front seat."

The day was filled with sun, memories, and laughter, mixed with childhood reflections and family regrets. It was one of those rare days when they caught some distant feeling of knowing they were still alive. The last stop on our tour was the ice cream parlor. As we stopped to park, Tom turned in his seat with a serious look on his face he declared, "Honey, I have plenty of ice cream at home. We're not far from my house." I was not aware until later that indeed his home was nearby.

As we entered the ice cream parlor, Tom encouraged everyone not to eat too much and save room for his party. I felt a deep sadness rise within me. I wanted to tell him that I couldn't take him home, but how does one explain to a parent that their adult child has terminated their emotional needs and desires. I tenderly patted his hand and tried to enter into idle conversation until the others finished their treat.

Upon leaving the parlor, Tom smiled and gently touched my hand. "Don't worry, I'll tell you where to turn." I smiled and drove on toward the nursing home. But about a mile from the parlor Tom's memory was triggered by a familiar sight causing him to react with anxious anger as he desperately tried to open the locked door. I quickly pulled the van into a convenience store to try and comfort him. I prayed that the story that was coming out of my mouth would come true. I grabbed his hand tightly as I explained the problem I was facing.

"Tom, I don't want to spoil your son's visit. I'm sure he's going to be taking you to visit your home tomorrow." He stared at me, for what seemed hours, then slowly smiled and relaxed back into his seat.

The next day Tom recalled nothing of the trip or my lie. But each day he seemed to withdraw a little further into himself. But why not? What else was left in life for Tom? He needed his family. Eventually, he was moved to the Alzheimer unit, which doubled the cost of his care. Did Tom suffer from Alzheimer disease? No. But that is another story.

~~~

Mary was a quiet, slim woman with no apparent physical handicaps. Standing inside the door to her room was a delicately designed pedestal four-feet high. Resting atop was an open guest book with three names and addresses dated from the previous year. It was the type of pedestal and guest book that might be placed in the parlor of a funeral home. I think, in many ways, Mary had died the day she was taken from her farm. She seemed to be waiting.

Quietly, she would sit erect with hands folded neatly in
~~~

her lap, eyes fixed to the tree outside of her window. Whether in her room or in the dining room, it was the same. Periodically, she would pick up a morsel of food from her plate, a drink of water, or sip of tea, a bite or two of bread, and she was finished.

She once explained the details concerning her son "running" her off of her farm. "He brought me to this hotel and now he and his family live on my farm. They got what they wanted. That's o.k. I'll just sit here and wait till they leave."

Several months later I began to notice that Mary had stopped eating. I was afraid it was the beginning of withdrawal. A few days later I decided to make a fruit bowl for her of strawberries and melon. She had become very weak, but was still able to get to the dining room.

On that bright, sunny day, I seated Mary by the dining room window with her bowl of fruit. She smiled, picked up a strawberry, and gently bit into the red beauty. I was so excited for her. We hugged and I ran to the nurse's station to share the good news. The nurse's aide greeted me and I told her that maybe they should keep Mary on a fruit diet because she was trying to eat.

"Well, honey, she'll probably do a lot better now that we got that denture out and cleaned it."

The aide proceeded to tell me that she had noticed "some kind of stuff" that looked like it was growing on Mary's gums. "I started looking real close and saw she had a partial denture. Nobody ever told me. It's not on her record. I looked. I've been here for four months and she has been here three years. It took two of us to get it out of her mouth. Honey, you have never smelled anything so bad when we got it out. Her mouth was rotten."

I stood looking at the aide in utter horror. I couldn't think of anything to say. I turned and went back to Mary and the bowl of fruit. She had eaten two strawberries, folded her hands in her lap and was sitting in her erect fashion — eyes fixed on the sky. As the days went by, Mary grew weaker contracting pneumonia and passed away soon after.

How could something as simple as a denture be overlooked? When a person is admitted to a nursing home they arrive with a physician's order regarding prescriptions, psycho-social problems, medical history, etc. The Admissions Director reviews the records with family members and passes them on to the "charge" nurse. Since Mary's denture had not been listed on her admittance records, the oversight would have been a shared error with the physician and Admitting Director.

My anonymous request to the Department of Health proved futile. They were working under a three month backlog of investigation requests, but promised to contact me once they made an investigation. I was never contacted and to my knowledge an investigation was never made.

~~~

Neglect by adult children is not always intentional. But unless an individual has been employed or resided in a nursing home, they can never have a complete
~~~

understanding of the loneliness that their loved ones experience. Separated from their family and the world outside, most residents simply "grin and bare it," while others find their refuge in various types of neurotic behavior.

While volunteering my services at a reputable, church funded nursing home, I was introduced to an amazing woman of 92 years. Pearl had graduated from a Washington, D.C. high school in 1918. Trained in social and secretarial skills, she found employment immediately as an assistant to a bookkeeper. The following year she met and married her husband, a veteran of World War I.

Pearl worked as a homemaker until tragedy struck in 1929 when her husband was killed in an accident, leaving her an unemployed widow with three small children at the onset of the Great Depression. One year later Pearl secured a secretarial position in the newly founded Veterans Administration where she was employed until her retirement in the mid-sixties.

She had decided to move to Texas to be near her daughter, where she spent several more years as an active participant in community affairs. But when her time came to readjust her lifestyle, her daughter – then 68 years – did not offer her home to Pearl. So, Pearl admitted herself to their church supported nursing home.

I hesitantly asked Pearl if she would rather be in a home environment. She looked at me as if she had to respond to a silly child's question.

"Well now, what do you think? Does this look like the way you would want to end your life?"

At that moment, the telephone rang. It was her daughter. She was arriving in an hour to take Pearl home for the weekend.

~~~

I am constantly amazed at the length of time that a person can endure emotional neglect. Patty was an overweight, petite woman in her 80th year. Physically, she was normal, but mentally, she had suffered periods of depression. Instead of treating the depression, because of her age, she was admitted to the nursing home.

Patty had one daughter who visited, maybe, twice a month. Throughout the duration of my employment, I tried tenderness, consistency in my room visits, art therapy, crafts, and entertainment, but nothing that I suggested or brought to Patty's room created a response or motivated the slightest smile.

She never participated in conversation other than to ask when her daughter would be visiting. Her daily routine was to move herself two feet over from the bed to the chair where she spent the day watching television. Although, she did not appear to become involved in any of the programming.

Several weeks before resigning my position, I noticed Patty had taken to walking back and forth in the hallway directly in front of her door. She had changed her daily pattern and unless the change in pattern is positive, it usually is a warning of mental and physical collapse. I reported her behavior change to my supervisor and tried to
~~~

use my skills to calm Patty. But, in my soul, I knew the problem and I knew Patty had no other choice but to "pass away." She had lived in limbo for three years. No visitors and a "too-busy" daughter.

A couple of days later I found Patty lying across her bed gasping for breath. Immediately, she was rushed to the hospital where she succumbed to pneumonia. Her daughter could not be reached. Ironically, Patty had displayed no signs of pneumonia. I remembered the metaphysical term for pneumonia was to feel that life was smothering and trapping you until you are unable to breath freely. How true that was for Patty.

~~~

It was common knowledge that Lewis had been a man of great wealth and accomplishments. But to Lewis, his greatest accomplishment was his healthy head of hair and mouth full of his own teeth. His jovial personality and gentleness won the hearts of staff and visitors.

Lewis was a strong, healthy man of 90 years when I first introduced myself to him and his ailing wife. Reva and Lewis were our lovebirds. Although blessed with good health and a clear mind, Lewis had entered the nursing home in order to remain with his wife. They shared the same room and bed for nine months before Reva quietly passed away in her sleep. Lewis had always held firm to the idea that he could keep her alive as long as he was next to her.
~~~

The morning that he awoke to discover her cold body was the beginning of the end for Lewis. His grief severely affected his appetite and in a month's time he had lost 15 pounds. The staff and I worked feverishly to create tempting dishes for Lewis over the following two weeks that followed. Step by step, morsel by morsel, we seemed to make progress, until, at last, we cheered as Lewis ate his first full meal.

When I arrived home that evening, I fixed a special sweet treat for Lewis. The next morning I hurried to his room to present him with a special gift box full of fudge. As I walked past the nurses station showing off my box of goodies for Lewis, I was informed that he had been taken to the dentist. His daughter had arranged for him to have his teeth pulled and replaced with dentures. The news hit me like an electric shock. *Was the woman insane,* I thought? I knew how much Lewis respected his only daughter. She had been a "change of life" baby and Lewis could not say enough about her beauty and brains. He would never protest her decision.

I knew I had to stop her. I rushed to the Administrator's office to plead with him to call the dentist. I knew by previous experience that it was hopeless to get immediate action from the health department. The only person with the authority to terminate the dental trip was the Administrator. But that would mean risking, a $4,000 dollar a month income. The conversation was put to a sudden halt when he made it clear that he would not interfere in family decisions.

Lewis survived his wife's death, but not the extractions

of his teeth. He hated the appearance of his dentures and the pain he silently bore wore deeper into his grief until Lewis would no longer eat anything. He simply stopped living and died. The death report claimed his death to be of "natural causes." But we all knew that there was nothing natural about it. There was nothing natural about a daughter that harbored such a strong unresolved issue that it would cause her to execute such a sadistic deed.

Part Four
To Be Sure

Some frightened soul,
who to end his own confusion
caused a million tears,
threw away a million moments
of tenderness, just to feel
the illusion of control.
What we are, is temporary,
but everything we do,
or do not do ... is forever.

Thousands of seniors every year are admitted to nursing homes after being diagnosed with Dementia. Dr. Nathan Billig, M.D., author of *To Be Old and Sad* and Associate Professor of Psychiatry at the Georgetown University Medical Center in Washington D.C., claims that twenty percent of Dementia cases are reversible. Dr. Billig has found that the causes of these symptoms that appear to be a form of Dementia are adverse effects of certain medications, depression, metabolic, and endocrine problems, certain nutritional abnormalities, and neurological conditions.

The family should insist on a complete mental and chemical evaluation of the patient and should never tolerate the notion that the symptoms of Dementia are a normal part of aging.

Leonard L. Heston, M.D., and Associate Scientist, June A. White of the University of Minnesota, researched and wrote, *Dementia (A practical guide to Alzheimer's*

Disease and related illnesses). The book explains that Alzheimer's, one of several types of Dementia, was noted to have several tests that could determine whether the individual was suffering from Alzheimer's, (or another type of Dementia), or suffered from a chemical imbalance. Medical science had established that a deficiency in hormones, vitamins, or electrolytes will cause abnormalities in the thinking processes.

Nursing homes rely completely on the physician's orders when admitting and placing the ailing elder in specific units. Families should realize that nursing homes are not in the business of nursing your family member back to health. Therefore, they have no motivation toward questioning the validity of a physician's diagnoses. The responsibility to question and demand to know all possibilities that could cause the problem is strictly on the shoulders of the family.

James F. Balch, M.D., and co-author of the 1990 publication, *Prescription for Nutritional Healing*, claims that all of the following problems can exhibit the same symptoms as Alzheimer's:

Hardening of the arteries; minor strokes (causing loss of brain tissue); Toxic reactions to drugs; small clots to the brain; advanced syphilis; Brain tumors; hypothyroidism; toxic metals in the body, (a hair analysis will determine if this is the problem).

Dr. Balch explained that there is a strong correlation between Alzheimer's disease and excessive amounts of bromine, calcium, sulfur, and silicon concentrated in the brain, (determined through autopsies of Alzheimer victims). The autopsies also revealed that the deficiencies were of boron, potassium, selenium, B12 and zinc. Dr. Balch now believes that it is quite possible that these results may suggest excessive amounts of aluminum in the diet, combined with a lack of several essential minerals, directly, or indirectly, predispose one to Alzheimer's disease. Aluminum pans are not the only culprit in the body's collection of aluminum. Dr. Balch lists the following items that are potentially hazardous aluminum derivatives:

A. Food additives
B. Douches (vinegar and water could substitute).
C. Antacids
D. Buffered aspirin
E. Anti-diarrheal preparations
F. Aluminum beverage and food containers

It is a long and tedious process to reach a legitimate determination on the type of Dementia present. As an Activity Director, it was my responsibility to know the medical and social history of each resident in my recreational therapy program. Many of which, had been diagnosed with Alzheimer's disease, or a specific type of Dementia. In the first stage of the Alzheimer's disease it is relatively impossible to distinguish the victims' actions from those suffering from a particular type of Dementia, or mental illness.

~~~
~~~

Georgia, an active woman of 76 years, displayed all the signs of a mild form of Dementia, but had been diagnosed with Alzheimer's, whereas, Flo, a woman four years Georgia's junior, sat in a semi-catatonic state. Her action or non-action was typical of many with advance stages of Alzheimer's disease. But Flo had been diagnosed with an undisclosed type of Dementia. Ironically, both women had developed their condition soon after the deaths of their husbands.

Georgia had been a resident of the nursing home for four years. But her personality had remained stable. She was talkative, cordial, and very active. Her memory spanned all stages of her life, but she could not recall five minutes or five days prior.

Flo had retired to the nursing home with her husband, six years before the term of my employment. Flo, like Lewis, had chosen to be with her ailing spouse, rather then live without him. When he died she slowly withdrew into herself. It was obvious that she was aware of everything around her, but chose to sit silently, watching.

My position allowed me access to approximately 400 medical histories and diagnosis of the entire nursing home population. During my term of employment I never discovered a chart with a treatment plan for mental illness, even though it was apparent that many of the residents suffered from a variety of phobias and neurosis as a result of traumatic events in their lives.

Two months after I began my employment, I included Georgia and Flo in an art program, which allowed them to paint flowers and landscapes. I discovered from Flo's family friend, that during the 40's, Flo had worked as a professional painter and designer. The day I brought her into the art room and laid out her paint and canvas was a day I would never forget. Her eyes welled with tears as sounds of "oohs" and "oh, oh" came between her hesitant touches from brush to paint. It was like watching a mother touch her newborn child for the first time.

Georgia, our presumed, Alzheimer's victim was excited with the prospects of producing a finished product to hang in her room. There was no hesitation for her. She picked up the brush with the ease of a child at play. And that was exactly how Georgia viewed the process. But for Flo, it was a part of her soul that had been misplaced and now found. She sat in front of her canvas for two classes before finding the courage to pick up the brush and paint. It had been years since she had expressed the two greatest loves of her life — her talent and the love for her husband.

After one month of art classes, Flo was talking in short sentences and dancing to her favorite tunes. Georgia had finished several child-like paintings, which she periodically carried to the dining room to "show-off" to the dinner crowd. The conclusion of this experiment lead me to believe that emotional illness, not Dementia or Alzheimer's disease was the dominating, unspoken, and untreated illness suffered by most residents. I believe that the lack of a correct diagnosis' for the elderly revolves around society's lack of respect for their probable worth in creating a treatment plan for a person who, most likely, has a limited time left to live.

Drug researchers (in the early nineties), at Southwestern Medical School in Dallas, Texas, would periodically advertise a need for Alzheimer's victims in *SR Texas*, a senior publication. The purpose was to test new drugs on willing victims. In 1992, Dupont Pharmaceutical Company used the school's researchers to test a drug that reversed or slowed the disease.

The study was heartbreaking to families and many of the researchers and assistants. It was a cruel test that required the withdrawal of the drug from further use at the close of the study period. At that time, Dupont sent the drug and the test results to the FDA for the long wait. But the participants of the test whose lives briefly returned to normal, awoke one day to find the experiment had ended, as well as the drug that brought their sanity.

One research assistant at the Southwest Medical School who wished to remain anonymous, regretted the withdrawal of the drug from the participants when their progress was so obvious. She also agreed that most physicians do not bother to test to find the type of Dementia an elder is exhibiting. Usually a diagnosis is based on the daily actions of the elder.

Tests are costly and most people feel the probability of the elder returning to a normal life is non-existent anyway. It is very possible that a person of 70 years may have 20 to 30 years of contributions to make to family and society. Is this not worth a little time and expense to bring an elder back to health and sanity?

In May of 1993, the Federal Drug Administration claimed to have the oldest U.S. Public Affairs employee.

Emil Corwin was a proud man of 90 years. He had been hired by the agency when he was 72 years. It would have been just as possible for Mr. Corwin to have had a reaction to a drug and diagnosed with Dementia one year before being hired by the FDA. The point being that people are worth testing and saving, if only for ten additional years. Books can be written, a child nurtured, a friendship renewed, a project completed, and a fear resolved.

My first knowledge of Alzheimer's disease came from text books and documentaries while attending a college course in Nursing Home Activity Director training. But, in no way did this knowledge prepare me for my first visit to an Alzheimer's Care Unit for advance stages. The first day I arrived on the job, my supervisor had suggested that I tour the unit with ten other new employees. She warned that my emotions would probably only allow me to stay a short time on my first visit. I laughed and assured her that I was not bothered by illness. "That's what they all say," she said sweetly.

As we approached the locked doors I began to feel nervous, but I attributed the discomfort to the idea of being behind locked doors. The thought of working within a secured environment seemed more frightening than the disease. But my opinion soon changed as the doors were opened to reveal men and women yelling, drooling, laughing and crying as if touched by demons. Some walked aimlessly down the hallway, while others were strapped in dining chairs repeating sentences or words for hours and sometimes *days*.

The scene seemed so familiar. I felt every nerve in my

body rise to the back of my neck. I could feel the confusion and mental pain. They seemed like characters in a movie I had seen as a child. A small woman nearby yelled obscenities to the large drooling woman seated next to her. Tears streamed down my cheeks as I stood politely smiling at her. My presence was as pointless to her as a store mannequin.

The tour group began moving through the unit — room to room, we said our "hellos" to these broken minds. As we walked back to the locked entryway, I remembered a movie watched as a child. It was called *The Snake Pit* and was produced in the 40's, depicting life in an insane asylum. Was it possible that the insane throughout past decades were merely victims of this cruel disease? This traumatic experience for the "first time" observer is what textbooks are unable to prepare within the visitor or family member.

The sorrow in viewing this regression is two-fold: mental and physical. The mental phases of regression seem to result in a conscious, as well as, subconscious explosion of traumas and emotions that were once buried deep in the psyche. The victim often relives the good times, as well as the bad or becomes "stuck" on a treadmill of images and words. The ease in which they will regress will depend on the person's personality, lifestyle, and family ties. These factors also determine how long the victim will stay in each phase.

Naomi Feil, ACSW, author and founder of "Validation Therapy," states, "Each human being is different and valuable, no matter how disoriented. Each stage of life has different goals. There is reason behind all behavior." Mrs. Feil's therapy revolves around the idea that "the old and diseased must reconcile with the living in order to prepare for dying." Early-learned emotional memories replace intellectual thinking in the diseased elderly. The idea is to validate what they are experiencing.

Alzheimer's Disease takes the elder through many physical and mental regressions – back, back, and back to the womb stage. Each stage of regression triggers a feeling that was once ignored or enjoyed. This is the factor that determines the speed in which the supposed disease will take control.

The atrocity of nursing home care for this disease is the lack of individual psychological care. The majority of Alzheimer's units admit only first or second stage victims, but few Medicaid nursing homes have an Alzheimer's unit. Religious/Denominational homes such as Baptist, Jewish and Presbyterian, offer individualized attention at a higher ratio than private pay homes.

The obvious professional planning and participation needed for each individual's mental and physical comfort and therapy, challenge the validity of state and federal laws on pre-admission screening. Since January 1, 1989, federal law states that facilities may not admit any person with serious mental illness, unless state approved. This law does not include Alzheimer's or related Dementia, as these are not classified as mental illness, under the Pre-admissions Screening and Annual Resident Review, (PASARR).

Robert L. Taylor, M.D., California State University,

discussed in his article, "Screening for Medical Referral," published in "Current Psycho Therapies," 4th Edition, by Raymond J. Corsini and Danny Wedding. Dr. Taylor explains how necessary, but difficult it is to discern psychological problems from organic psychological disorders. He claims that anxiety, depression, paranoia, and obsessive-compulsive disorders are often, the products of psychological conflict.

A list of these medical conditions include viral encephalitis, head injuries, brain tumors, petit mal epilepsy, hyper-calcemia, drug intoxications, heart disease, and diabetes. Prescription and non-prescription drugs are the number one cause of organic mental disorders, according to Dr. Taylor.

Alzheimer's disease is claimed by the medical profession to be an organic mental disorder, but with many of the same symptoms attached to psychological problems. It has been established that statistically people 55 and beyond have a higher risk for organic mental disorders. Psychiatric hospitalization for people 55 years into experience and beyond have an organic basis. Chronic physical disease combined with several types of medications establishes the increased risk of adverse mental and emotional reactions.

The emotional drain of working with Alzheimer's disease, as well as other types of Dementia, and disease, puts the nursing home nurses and activity employees at risk for "burn out" after one year of employment. The state and federal habits of overlooking Dementia and Alzheimer's disease as a mental illness is ludicrous.

Medical science has proven that it is difficult to distinguish the difference between organic anxiety, depression, paranoia, and obsessive-compulsive disorder vs. the same mental disorder as a result of psychological conflict.

The National Citizens' Coalition For Nursing Home Reform has failed to address this issue. The questions then arise as to why nursing homes are allowed to operate Alzheimer/Dementia units without a high ratio of experienced psychiatric attendants and nurses aides. Is it because 95 percent of the occupants are 70 years and older?

We must, at some point, realize that nursing homes are not in the business of "wellness" therapy or pre-admission screening to determine whether how to solve a mental disorder that has lead to an organic or psychological conflict. Alzheimer's units and nursing homes are merely a form of "holding tank" until death-do-they-part. Home care for individuals who are perceived to be irreversible Dementia or Alzheimer's victims is the kindest form of care. This, of course, depends on the strength of love and respect within the family unit.

A 1980's movie release entitled, "Folks," starring Tom Selleck, centered around the plight of a young family man and the problems and traumas he incurred while trying to fit an aging mother and a father with Alzheimer's disease into his own family lifestyle. The movie was written as a dramatic comedy with a warm insight into the lengths some children will go to for the good of the family unity. The message given through the trials and tribulations of trying to care for a family member with Alzheimer's disease was the respect for human life — in any condition. The story closed with the son's solution to the problem being a country home for his family, and a trailer for his parents. Dad was then free to wander through the country fields — safe at last.

Part Five
Keeping The Reason Alive

I think in term of multiplicities,
conquests unseen, marches to nowhere,
the journey, the test, a vision quest.

A traveler I am, a bird, a light,
a place in the sun, a night of fun.

I find it right to find myself amidst the clouds,
of lavender lights and fearless flights.

I'm told, I'm bold, a story untold,
a beggars banquet, an otter, a potter.

Could be, I'm me,
and what would that be,
to be the me I want to be?

A little young, a little old,
a little to little, and I would be cold.

So what do you do, when you are you,
and you know it's too late to hesitate?
So as you see, I have to be me,
to carry on … sing my song,
in opulent multiplicities.

The mystery of the personal quality … genes, or determination that drives some families, or individuals, to ignore the mental confines of age, is profiled in the lives of the following ageless individuals. It is a priceless gift to encourage a loved one to continue their own self expression. Many individuals, labeled by others as "old", do not see the continuation of their lifestyle as being a choice of "do or don't." It is simply, their own personal, on-going, process of living their desires and values. And as the years mount, they seem to be oblivious to wrinkles or aching bones. Their goal is to live, laugh, love and express their unique talents and personality in themselves and those around them — at any cost.

The fact is that there is nothing unique about those who live their life without acknowledging age. It is normal and our God given right. Only limited thought, born of fear, can stop this right of freedom.

An example of a family's gift of purpose came from my father's side of the family. My grandmother passed away in 1946, a period when nursing homes were virtually non-existent. Grandmother was a buxom, pioneer woman who had braved her early motherhood traveling from Missouri to Oklahoma in a covered wagon with eight children. During the Great Depression she and Grandfather lived in a one room prairie house farming red sandy soil to feed their family. Longevity was not her fate and her passing came after 65 years of experience.

I was seven years at the time, but I remember the love

and understanding that was executed in helping Grandfather readjust his lifestyle. He was "Gentleman Jim" to those who knew him, born James Valentine Risner in the year 1876. Grandfather was a never-ending storybook concerning the wild days of his early life. Covered wagons, trappers, gamblers, and outlaws. I never tired of listening to him tell of the day when he watched Jesse James ride through his hometown of Thayer, Missouri.

Because of Grandfather's love of conversation, my father and his three brothers, and four sisters decided it was out of the question for him to spend the remainder of his life on a remote farm. So, with the help of his children, a new wardrobe, and a monthly allowance from each, he embarked on a ten year adventure of travel and an endless flow of conversation.

His children were located in areas from Detroit, Michigan to Oklahoma, so he traveled by bus to the home of each son and daughter spending a month to two months annually with each adult child. The grandchildren knew the time of year that Grandfather would arrive and we all breathlessly awaited this unique character who would tell us the secrets of life along with stories that could only be found in a Zane Gray novel.

Grandfather was an avid reader with only a fifth grade education. But name any subject and he could tell us all about it, along with his positive and negative viewpoints. Grandfather was never shy about admitting his lack of education, but would quickly add, "In my day the fifth grade was like a high school education these days." I was never sure what that meant, but as a child I decided that the children in his time must have been of a higher intellect then we were.

"Gentleman Jim," the last generation of the American pioneer, projected an image of youth that planted a seed in my soul forever allowing me to grow as a person, not a number. Grandfather passed away ten years after the onset of his new lifestyle. It was the day after he had danced and sang at my 16th birthday. He passed-on while waiting to get a haircut — laughing and telling jokes — the end was quick.

~~~

Molly is an 84 year Washington resident, and avid gardener. She won her battle over cancer and ignored the doctor's orders to refrain from the strain of maintaining an award winning flower garden. Molly projects a true pioneer spirit that she attributes to her early life as a resident in the wilds of Alaska.

Upon attaining 65 years of earthly life, she and her sister purchased a ship constructed in 1935. The project began as a restoration project, developing into their residence for five years. Her sister mastered the mechanics of keeping the engine operating, while both mastered the art of navigation. During the five years the two women made frequent trips to Alaska and islands throughout the Pacific Northwest.

The fairytale life ended for Molly when a scuba diving
~~~

accident took her sister's life. Molly was 70 years in experience when she lost her best friend. But she was determined to stay as close to the ocean as possible. She sold the ship and purchased a beach house on an island off the coast of Washington state.

"Life, to me, is about going on and experiencing new adventures." Molly's love for flowers opened new challenges when she decided to take up watercolor painting. Now she has many reasons to arise in the mornings. "Life is an on-going adventure of unfinished business and I want to get up in the morning to see how much of it I can get done — to feel the excitement of a new flower or a completed painting. Age has nothing to do with my life. I have always been a free spirit. What else are we here for, if not to find a reason to get up in the morning?"

~~~

Mom Brown has lived 85 years. She has lived in the same house since 1945. The small boned woman is a mere, four-feet, eleven-inches tall, weighing 98 pounds, but can still swing a hammer and paint the interior of her home.

"This neighborhood is considered a historical district now. I guess that means me too. I remember my husband bought this house for seven thousand dollars. I have never wanted to move. I had enough of moving when I was a child. I'm tough, but I like to be tough in one spot. I guess I got my survival spirit from my mother. She was a traveling minister during the Great Depression years. She
~~~

was 96 when she died. The most determined woman I have ever seen.

"There was five of us kids and we lived in St. Paul. My father worked for a good paying company so we had a nice house and a happy life. Then mother found her 'calling' in religion. My father was not a religious man, but a good man. But mother decided to save the world. She took us kids and left father behind. I remember living in a tent — going from city to city and church to church. I guess, that's why I hate traveling — leaving my house. We finally stopped traveling when we came to Texas. I was in grade school and that's where I met my lifelong best friend. We have done everything together over the years. Seventy, to be exact.

"I have raised my three children in this house and outlived two husbands and a couple of boyfriends. I guess this house is my anchor. It holds my memories and needs my constant attention. I'm always fighting with it. Something always needs fixing or painting. I hate waiting on people to do things for me, so I just do it. Oh, I've had my moments when I wanted to give-up. Like when Missy, my dog of 13 years, died. And when my brother was found dead. It's watching people and things leave your life that is so hard. I have lived here for 65 years now, and nothing is the same — little by little, the places where I shopped and went out dancing have all been torn down. The only thing that I can count on not to change is my house and my yard. That's what keeps me young. My children keep wanting me to move in with them, but then I would have nothing to take care of. Who wants to just sit and be old. That's what "old" means to me—just sitting with nothing important to take care of.

"Oh, I don't go out to bars anymore. Who would I dance with? I have tried dating a few guys my age, but their too grumpy and don't want to dance, so I'll keep looking. I always liked younger guys anyway."

~~~

David is 78 years, and a retired English teacher.

"Well, I decided to retire at 65 and buy this beach house. I sat, walked, pounded a few nails, and told myself I was lucky to have time to think, but then the thinking started working against me. I had played the piano all my life and so I decided to give piano lessons. But that was teaching again and I was tired of teaching. I was always a fanatic about keeping my piano tuned.

"One day it dawned on me that I could start a piano tuning business. My wife is an invalid and needed something to do, so we devised a system where she would take the calls and make the schedule. Well, the business grew quite rapidly, and it has turned out to be fulfilling for both of us. I meet new people and stay busy and she has a sense of worth … a reason to wake up in the morning. She has now decided to write our family history. It seems that purpose in our life breeds more purpose. Now we enjoy our waterfront home even more, but only in our spare time."
~~~

~~~

Fran was 97 years young when I met her. Her home is a three-room cabin nestled on the edge of an island forest in Washington state. At 97, Fran continues to tend her garden and feed the chickadees that run excitedly across the edge of her deck.

In 1966, Fran and her husband bought their dream property with the intentions of building their small retirement home. Six months later, Fran's husband and best friend, passed away. His sudden death left her with a major decision that she viewed as a crossroads in her life. It was approaching winter on the small island and Fran had planned to have the cabin built by Spring.

Funeral expenses had depleted the funds allocated to hire the labor needed to build the cabin. She knew there was only one way to make her dream come true. She would have to build it herself. She contacted a carpenter on the island to tell him her plan. He laughed and told her she would never be able to build it without help. After much confrontation and assurance that he would be paid, he agreed to lay the foundation and construct the frame.

It was bitter cold and the November winds and rain had arrived. Fran pitched her tent and began her work. She completed the exterior walls and roof of her cabin late that March, after her 68th birthday.

The first time that I walked through her accomplishment, I ask her how she had learned to build a house. "If you can sew, you should be able to build a house." Fran related to
~~~

me that she had always had a determined spirit, since her college experience. Women were not allowed in college design courses in 1916. But with the help of a father with social status, she was allowed entry.

She laughed while sharing her story of being a class outcast. "The professor and the men in class ignored me, always whispering behind my back. But I didn't care. I remained focused and finished my courses at the top of the class. I never gained acceptance with them, even though I proved my ability. I felt like I was going through the same thing all over again when I was building my cabin. Friends of the carpenter, who laid the foundation, would drive by while I was working and tell me that I should give it up and let a man do it."

Fran is still amazed that she has lived such a long time. "I thought that I would only live to enjoy it for a couple of years." I ask her why she would want to go through such hardship if she was only expecting to live a few years more. "Because they told me I would never get it done."

~~~

A renewal of life comes in many forms, and it is not always what is considered socially acceptable, as in the case of 66 year young, Laura Jo. "Well, my husband died right after we bought this new home. So here I sat in a new house — paid for — no worries, living on my social security. But I was lonely. Oh, I had friends, but all they did was complain about aches and pains and their age.
~~~

"Then one day I was buying some plants at a nearby nursery where I met a young man. Oh, *I* say young. As it turned out, he was 46. But at the time, I was 60 years old. Well, *I* say "old," but I didn't feel old. Well, anyway, he started asking me questions about flowers, and telling me about his yard. We just hit it off. We ended up going for lunch and he ask if he could come and see my flower garden, sometime. Oh, my God! When he started coming over for regular visits I thought my friends and family were going to call the police on him. Everyone just knew he was out to do something bad. Well, he had more money and property than I did, so that eliminated that theory for everyone. They finally had to accept the fact that he just plain liked to be with me.

"Well, we had five years of heaven together. I never played and laughed so much in my life. He asked me to marry him a couple of times, but I just laughed at him. I still remember the day he told me he had cancer. The end for him was a sweet time for us and I can always be in peace knowing I was his comfort in the end. That little "stink" left me his property in a Will. I couldn't believe it. His family knew how much he loved me, so they didn't even try to fight it.

"That was almost a year ago. I'm not lonely anymore. I have such great memories from our five years that I just smile all the time. He gave me a new sense of myself. He made me realize that I am as young as I want to be. I am not recommending that all older women go out and find a younger man. My Randall was a special person that saw past the physical and brought out the playful spirit in me.

It was just one of those relationships that cannot be explained. It came at a time that we both needed it. Now, I do a lot of things that I never use to do before he came along … like sleeping in the raw."

~~~

Blackjack Jimmy was 98 years old when I met him. A "black" musician, (he said he wasn't from Africa and was just *plain* black). Jimmy would shuffle his feet along, leaning on his shiny chrome walker until he was safely in place, standing regally, in front of the nightclub stage.

Jimmy put all the energy and breath he had saved for the month in that one blues song. Beads of sweat would pop and run down his glowing face. He swayed and rocked back and forth while holding to his chrome walker. But, to Jimmy, all the pain and exhaustion was worth that one trip a month to sing as he did in the peak of his career. When the song was over, he was quickly ushered to a nearby chair.

The applaud and whistles, patrons gathering at his table — ladies giving him hugs. This was Jimmy's reason for living one more month. He never knew if it would be his last song, so he gave it his "all." Jimmy Jack had lived and sang with the best original Blues singers in the business. He had seen the "Negro" (he still held to the old way of referring to African Americans), community that he was born into, slowly become an area of expensive historical homes and offices, splattered with fancy venues.
~~~

Jimmy didn't have a fear, about his color. He only knew that music was his purpose and he knew he was good at what he loved. It didn't matter where, or who he sang to — it was all about the amount of "soul" that he could give to others.

~~~

Fred was 82 years experienced and lived in an 80-year-old house that he purchased during World War II. Fred, now alone in the two story house, spent his waking hours patching and painting it inside and out. He thought nothing of climbing a ladder and patching the roof. Nor did two heart attacks seem to have an effect on his determination to stay busy.

His wife, 25 years his junior, had divorced him long ago. They had remained friends, but her constant nagging to sell his home and move to a nursing home brought him more misery than did his ill health.

Fred grew up on an east Texas farm and worked as a truck mechanic from the age of 18 until he retired at 70. Working was Fred's life, and that is how he wanted to leave this world — working. Ironically, Fred was the "apple" of every elderly woman's eye in the neighborhood. He repaired their cars, washing machines, porches, flat tires, and seemed to have no limits in the extent of his handyman abilities.

Cakes, pies, rainy day lunches and warm dinners awaited Fred each week from the ladies he had saved from
~~~

some mechanical demon. Fred's simple advice to living was, "Life is about fixing what is broken. And I'm not talking just about things. We gotta keep on fixin' the way we think, too. There is a lot of things to fix for everyone. When you stop 'fixin' you stop livin'."

~~~

There is a distinct difference in the social concept that surrounds the age factor in rural areas, as opposed to metropolitan areas. In the great Northwest, pioneers still thrive in their 90th year. Many fend for themselves on forest land they have maintained since the 1930's. Retiring is something one does at the end of the day. The struggles, the challenges to survive in the rural and mountain area are never questioned. It is a way of life and it continues until the end.

Ned was 96 years along in his growth when I met him. I was working in a small law office 35 miles from the Cascade foothills. One day he appeared at our office door — small thin man carrying a tall thin walking stick. It was a sight I will never forget. Ned was dressed in tan cotton trousers that had been cut to fit his leg length. Over time the cut had frayed and become a fringe of various lengths of thread. His suspenders had been adjusted to high pulling his pants above his ankles. This comical creation was complimented by a green checked flannel shirt and a baseball cap that seemed to have had a life of it's own.

Ned lived alone except for a
~~~

caretaker that lived in a small cabin on his property. He decided that he wanted to change his Will and Power of Attorney, leaving his property and assets to his 62 year nephew. During the course of our interview I was amazed to find that he did not need glasses to see the paperwork. Nor did he have any problems with relating short-term, as well as long-term events, business goals and plans for the future.

I also discovered that day that Ned and I owned property less than half a mile from each other. I was thrilled. It was a golden opportunity to visit with an area legend. In the next two years that followed our first meeting, our visits developed into a mutual respect and trust. There was often a quiet resolve about him. I never pushed Ned to become familiar with his life and often our weekly visits consisted of a mixture of silence and a short exchange of questions and answers.

On rare occasions, Ned would voluntarily share vivid stories of his life as a Logger from the 1920's into the 60's. These were the special days and I was honored to sit by his old wood stove listening to the last of America's mountain pioneers.

It was hard for me to imagine this tiny man as a Logger. I had met many of them in the area and their strength and size seemed to be the requirement for the industry. But, his size had been an asset. He could climb the two and three hundred foot trees easier than the big guys. Trees had to be "topped" before they were cut down, and Ned could scurry faster and higher.

His major accomplishment was to have survived and

flourished in a territory where money and education was non-existent. Ned managed to work as a logger and save enough by 1939 to buy a humble home on 38 acres surrounding a small lake. Today the property is worth an estimated $500,000 thousand dollars. But this wasn't the end of Ted's accomplishment.

One cold rainy afternoon we sat looking out across his beautiful lake. Conversations with this pioneer revealed that he had saved and invested wisely.

He wanted to have money for emergencies. But costly emergencies never came. At 98 years, his total worth was near one million dollars. He lived as humbly as he did in 1939.

What keeps Ned alert and alive? He claims his secret is to make sure he keeps control over his own life. "Never give your 'control' over to another." In a recent discussion with him about his life and money he spoke in earnest to me.

"I'm at the stage that I don't want to be alone, but I don't want anyone comin' in and trying to take care of me, either. What I have worked hard to get keeps me in control of my life. I'm leaving it to my nephew, but it won't mean the same to him. I proved something to myself. Life was hard back then. Any money I made I kept it. I hunted deer and birds — got my own food and water. The hard work kept me movin' and if your not movin', you'll die."

At this writing, Ned is still living life his way. He often talks of selling his property and starting over. The spirit to recreate himself is still well and thriving in Ned.

~~~

Faye lost both legs to diabetes. She lives near her daughters, in a humble two bedroom home nestled at the base of a tree-covered mountain. Chickens gather across her porch each morning waiting for her wheelchair to appear at the door with their daily dose of feed.

Faye continues to care for herself and her home, with a little help from loved ones dropping in for daily visits. She married young and was a farmer's wife the majority of her life. What is this rural spirit that stands as strong as the trees and mountains? Do the vibrations of the natural wonders infuse the inhabitants with a strength that is lost to the cities?

A woman of 75 years, living alone. No bitterness or pity dimmed the gleam in her eyes. Like a fallen tree downed by the ravages of wind, her fate was accepted. But fallen or not, nothing is wasted in the rural areas of the Great Northwest.

Fallen trees become the God mother that holds tightly to new seedlings. Clutching her, they grow from her nourishment and the strength of the living organism that no longer stands erect in the sun. Faye had no regrets. Her daughters grew up under the wings of a mother who taught them the importance of the dignity that comes from self reliance. They could never imagine their mother being any other way.
~~~

Part Six

The Fallacy of Decline Lies In The Alchemy of Knowing

It is apparent that the belief in aging, as a state of decline, is an outdated fallacy which the majority of medical doctors continue to hold true as a "natural" deterioration process within the physical body. Of course, this makes a diagnosis much easier when ignoring the root thought or collection of life issues that put into motion the release of toxins, and general closed circuit malfunctions that cause deterioration. We have advanced to a stage of technical enlightenment, while ignoring the power of healing creative energy we hold within. This knowledge is known and accepted by scientists, physicians, clergy and prophets since the beginning of history. Now we come face to face with a fallacy that has become a detriment to the American Society and the human spirit.

My never- ending story in the trial and error of my personal demonstration of the illusion of aging has often instilled, in me, the feeling of charging through a battlefield hearing nothing but my own "rebel yell," as I run towards the enemy of ignorance. But, often, when the smoke clears and I find myself still standing … the glory sings inside as I wave my mental and spiritual flag of freedom.

Since my 50th year of experience on this earth my journey to prove my agelessness has entered phases of mild insanity, determined courage, headstrong adventure, and a constant child-like flirtation with fate. But above all, my life continues to stretch my imagination to the limitless possibilities that are open to me as long as I let go of programed aging restrictions, imposed by current practitioner's of medicine who treat, only, from a physical perspective. Ironically, this type of practice has changed very little from the medieval medical community.

The job of today's medical doctor should be to sustain the physical well being as a support measure while working in conjunction with a psychotherapist, and, or, metaphysical healer. Finding the answer to an ailment or disease must begin with the thought process, life issues and repressed pain and sorrow. The psychotherapist, physician and metaphysical healer would be an ideal trinity in propelling the discovery and healing process.

One of my favorite quotes comes from Hippocrates — *"Disease is not an entity, but a fluctuating condition of the patient's body, a battle between the substance of disease and the natural self-healing tendency of the body."*

I ask you, "What causes this natural healing tendency within the body?" The body could not heal without the desire of the mind to heal. Now, let's play a game with Hippocrates, replacing a couple of words in his quote.

Afflicted thoughts are entities causing fluctuating conditions in the patients body, resulting in a battle between the substance caused by the afflicted thought and the innate desire of the mind to heal.

Letting go of "familiar ground" is the first step in opening the doors to a new understanding of life. Familiar ground can be anything in our life we are tired of doing, being, or not doing or being. It is the ground of unquestioned acceptance. It is a zone that zaps our inspiration and leaves us drained, bored, restless, angry, or full of regrets. It is a space where life seems to have no spiritual connection to who, and what we proclaim to be, and so we find that we are nothing more than cows grazing in the pasture of time. In my case, I think it was all of the above.

In 1999, I escaped the pollution, noise and boredom of city life. My dream was to continue writing in the mountains of Western Washington. A single woman blooming with 60 years of city life experience, living in a mountain forest? Family and friends were doubtful that I would adapt to such a change of environment at "my age." But the thought of a new life left me breathless with excitement. I felt it was an opportunity to demonstrate my belief that life has no end to growth and excitement.

I cannot tell you the secret of letting go of the idea of aging. I have never allowed myself to think of it as part of my existence, except through the confusion of watching others accept it readily and insisting that I had no choice but to do the same. My determination to be myself without the stigma of age attached, has led me up and down many roads, and to one ultimate awakening. Living life, in the spirit of adventure without worry of what others think, is the truly the fountain of eternal youth.

If you are over 50, and socialize, exclusively, with people who are in the same stage of life experience, you will travel, eat and sleep cheaper than the rest of the world, but does it really fulfill the spirit within? Is it worth trapping yourself within the confines of a number, or label?

The senior citizen (coupon collecting) status has become an outdated concept of an American Dream that desperately needs re-VISION. The average american 50 and over is rarely considered a "shut-in," but they quietly accept the idea of being socially and economically "shut-out." Where is this voice of America that is now a majority? What will become of a nation that embraces the concept of decline?

The metaphysical New Age movement has accomplished wonders in revealing the ageless qualities awaiting each Human Being. But who will join us in our dance of Light? It matters not! It is your Light — your freedom and you will be right in step with the world's great metaphysical minds. You are not alone.

Am I rebelling against our accepted view of aging and decline? Yes! I did not make the rules that label humans as "over the hill" when they reach a certain number of birthdays. And it is not a law of the land that I accept such an insult.

The focus on Aging in our society has many faces, and presents our social scheme with a tidy way to give all Americans over 40, a quiet plan to "snuff" out their spirit. The problem is that the majority of society is now over 45. The American Dream has changed leaving a social problem for most Americans. Our outdated American Dream of a perfect life retiring in a little pink house with no financial problems has become extinct, but we have not changed our social schematics to fit the current reality.

There is an inner peace in being free of social convictions. It begins with realizing that you are not a statistic or label. Birthdays are not to be hidden or dreaded if celebrated for what they are: *a celebration of the gift of "life."* We are made in the image and likeness of God our Creator. God is Spirit, therefore we are Spirit. There are no time limits as to what we can experience or how much we can learn.

The journey begins with the realization that you are the only one that can experience your own unique adventure. You cannot experience your journey through the lives of your parents, children, neighbors or friends. In order to continue our growth and to feed our spirit, we must find the courage to create new ways and new adventures for ourselves. This is our heritage.

One morning, I was standing at the top of a flight of stairs that I had tumbled down the week prior. Suddenly, memory of my Aunt's death gave me a warning signal. My Aunt had passed-on shortly after her 75th birthday. She was a beautiful woman who maintained her appearance with as much style and care as she had in her early years. Her ability to present herself as ageless continually allowed her to secure work in the management field. At the time of her passing she was managing a large condominium resort in Houston.

Aunt Flo had conquered age limitations in the business world, but not socially. Underneath her bubbling personality boiled a bitter brew of anger. Her social life with mixed age groups had been full until her late fifties. But, one by one, to her dismay, she watched her friends retire into lives surrounding senior groups and activities. She refused to be labeled "old" and eventually viewed the business world as her only substitute for social interaction with all ages.

One bright sunny day, Aunt Flo stepped out of her office door to cross the parking lot. On the second step down she lost her footing, falling head first onto the pavement. She was rushed to the hospital, where she lingered for three days in a coma before passing-on. Two weeks before her Passing she had called me asking me to visit. She wanted to do something exciting. I was getting prepared for an art exhibit and couldn't get away.

As I stood at the top of the stairway that morning, I suddenly understood why I had lost my balance the week before. I had been involved with a man 22 years my junior for two years and had become worried that he would leave me for a mutual friend of ours that was in her 30's. My fear turned to anger, bringing me to the decision that I had put myself in a "no win" situation. I had turned my anger onto myself that fateful morning and for one second of angry thought I didn't care where I walked. But, the Angels had other plans for me. No broken bones — just a rude awakening.

The fall was merely an extension of my thought of falling out of the relationship. I had already fallen in my mind. My belief system was again being challenged and I was angry. Suddenly the thought of women with less life experience than myself, created the indignation that I was losing him to a number.

The fall seemed to have awakened in me visions of my Aunt Flo. I realized that she had limited herself socially by believing that she was socially segregated. She accepted it and her anger instilled in her a lack of balance to her life. The metaphysical approach to life is to start with thought of issues and fear to find the reason for accidents or disease. The answer was apparent.

The following day I decided that I would continue to see

the my friend and lover with the knowledge that all things end on this earth.. Maybe I would outgrow him and maybe he would outgrow me. Isn't that the same possibility of couples in their early 20's or in their late 90's? Life has no guarantees, no matter what social norms want to dictate.

To let go of America's concept of aging, you must first let go of society's concepts of what your actions, dress, and hairstyle, should be at a certain age. Once you succeed in believing you are ageless don't expect others to see you as ageless. You must first prove it to yourself before others will follow. It is your own spiritual freedom that you are setting free.

I have often found it is sometimes uncomfortable for others to watch an experienced man or woman entering into a younger social bracket. Especially if they are successful in gaining the attention of the opposite sex. Letting- go of the illusion of age is a journey of growing towards your inner Light. It is about discovering the *Real You* ...the *God You* that lives forever eternal without a number. The fun part is that you will often be met with curiosity, and eventually, respect. There is not a class or school that teaches a certain way to act and feel to find an ageless life, or lifestyle. You must create your own magic.

I recently experienced a man of 35 years, an ex-star football player that could not touch his toes, even though he attended the local health club three times a week. His excuse was that he was just getting "old." When you become in- tune with the metaphysics of growing without a number you will suddenly discover the amazing fact that people seem to want to grow old. They look for it — talk about it — live for it, until finally, the body and mind obey. It is also an escape from the responsibility of working towards your highest potential, due to a lack of self esteem.

Once you begin to lose thought of your life beginning and ending within the confines of a group of numbers, you will discover that you somehow become ageless to those considered old, or young. I have often sat in a group of people with less life experience than I and listened to them talk about their expectations of physical problems when reaching 60. I became acutely aware that, not only did they discount me in being among the age group they were discussing, but they seemed to discount me as being part of any age group. I was merely part of the personality of the group — no more and no less. Mission, accomplished!

There was a time when I had achieved the 45th over the hill "mark." I looked great, but I was falling apart, physically and emotionally. It never entered my mind that the problem was age. I knew I was reacting to all the dramas and traumas that had exploded in my life within the past five years. Two divorces in five years and the loss of a popular television show had stripped me of my spirit. It was the "could have been — should have been — and wanted to be," sickness that I had never taken the time to work through on a mental or spiritual basis.

Doctors, neighbors and friends viewed my extreme weight loss and mental disorder as menopausal, but I knew I was in spiritual trouble … the physical reaction was merely the result of my denial of emotional pain. It had to come out in some way.

We are humans, full of emotions, not age. In order to

stay mentally and physically "at play" with our self, we must constantly face, and release issues. This is the ingredient that keeps the "brittle" out of our bones and the spirit like a playful child. This is the magic of agelessness.

Author's Note

One of the great anxieties of life in America stems from a socially imposed time factor that is accepted in mass, without question. This accepted time factor holds us in the grips of anxious and mad ambition until our monetary goals are reached by our 30th, or 45th year of life. If we have not achieved the monetary American Dream within this time period, a personal crisis begins for many believing they are out of time … over the hill. This social time factor sets the stage for physical and mental decline.

I was once reminded by a group of university students that people past their 40th year of life are not the only ones affected by this illusion of time vs. achievement. The following statement made by a first year university student will give you insight into the "setting of the American stage," wherein the "illusion of age" becomes the mark of some unseen beast. This beast appears to rule over our mortal and spiritual success or failure in America.

"We are trying to find majors in college that we feel are going to determine our entire life. We also try to finish college as quick as we can rather than submerging ourselves in the cultural changes and mental, physical and spiritual growth that should be more prevalent.

We are hurrying through life in order to achieve greatness (money, career, family, etc.). I think my age group is less worried about our current age number, but extremely worried about the age number at which we are suppose to have achieved the goals we set for ourselves, so early in life." M.H. Southern Methodist University

We, as a nation, must claim our right to live as a human beings and not as actors trying out for a part, living in fear that we will be turned away for being or appearing too "old" or young. A change in the way we think of time and the word "old" can begin by disassociating yourself and your view of others with age identity based on a number.

I have discovered that it is much easier to program a child to realize that life is their very own creation and that creation is called *experience* rather than *age, aging* or *old.*

My next door neighbor once asked my small granddaughter, "How old are you honey?" Isabella quickly looked at me with a big grin and declared with pride, "I have six years of experience now." How much more beautiful it is to acknowledge yourself as a time traveler rather than a victim of time.

Seaon Ducoté

Printed in the United States
21462LVS00001B/69

9 781413 701630